SO YOU WANT TO BE A VEGETARIAN?

A Step-by-step Guide to a Plant-Based Diet

Jordan A. DeLoach

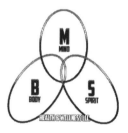

M.B.S. Health & Wellness L.L.C.
Southfield, MI

SO YOU WANT TO BE A VEGETARIAN?
A Step-by-step Guide to a Plant-Based Diet

Copyright © 2016 by Jordan A. DeLoach

Published by:
M.B.S. Health & Wellness L.L.C.
Southfield, MI 48033

ISBN 978-0-6926452-9-1

Cover by: Aija Monique Butler at ambbranding@gmail.com

Interior design by: interiorbookdesigns.com

Acknowledgments

First and foremost, I would like to thank the divine intelligence that has endowed me with the knowledge and wisdom to bring forth this work and the many other pieces I have created.

I want to thank my parents Anthony and Kimberley DeLoach for everything they have done thus far in helping me reach my goals in my adulthood and my adolescence, I would not be the man I am today without them. I would also like to thank them for their indirect inspiration that prompted me to step into vegetarianism and ultimately a vegan lifestyle-love you both!

Thanks to my sister Adrienne and my nephew Jaylen Napier for the love and support.

Thank you Avriele (April) Williams, you have been a major supporter in my life and very influential in keeping me focused on getting the book done.

I also have to thank Lakelia "Byrd" and Moe for all the knowledge and support and especially

Byrd for all of her genius in helping me with the book-glad to call you family.

I have to thank my brother from another Djuan Graves for the company logo and every other art piece done for me.

Thank you to everyone who has supported me on my health journey.

Thank you all.

Foreword

It is well known that a plant-based diet, whether vegetarian or vegan, is the most profound road to a healthy way of living today. It has been proven time and time again that a plant-based diet can prevent, and in many cases reverse some acute and chronic diseases, help with weight loss, and increase energy. Transitioning to a vegetarian diet can be a smooth transition for some yet difficult for others, it all depends on the individual – each experience is different. The goal with this book is to aide in making the transition as simple and stress-free as possible. The guide that will be laid out here is straight-forward and easy to follow. I realize reversing a habit many of us have had for our entire lives can take a good-deal of effort and energy so there's no need to make it even more complicated.

You've heard friends, family, and entertainers talk about how they regained and evolved their health by going vegetarian, now let's investigate how they did it!

Table of Contents

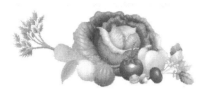

Foreword ix

A New Beginning 1

   The Link between Red/Processed Meat and Cancer.........3

   Now or Never..4

Chapter One - What is a Vegetarian....................................... 9

   Vegan vs. Vegetarian...9

   Benefits of a Vegetarian Diet...11

   How Eating Meat is Affecting You, Spiritually 13

   The Vegetarian Myth...15

Chapter Two - The Elimination Process 19

   Transitioning 19

   Cravings 23

Chapter Three - Becoming a Complete Vegetarian 29

   Critics..32

   Stick with It..33

   Health Benefits 34

Chapter Four - Shopping for Fruits and Veggies................39

   Eating at Restaurants..40

Meal Creativity 40

Jucing/Smoothies 41

Chapter Five - The Final Steps 45

Exercising to Increase Benefits 46

Becoming a Vegan...47

Vitamins and Supplements...................................49

You've Made a Big Step...50

5-Day Meal Plan 53

Appendix I...55

Appendix II - More Vegetarian & Smoothie Recipies 65

Notes..83

A New Beginning

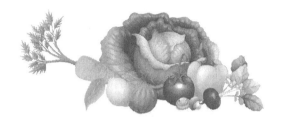

In today's industrialized society where chickens, cows, fish, and pigs, are raised and slaughtered in masse as a means of meeting the ever-growing demand of a population addicted to the consumption of animal flesh, many people have awakened to the reality of the matter and are searching for an alternative. The number of individuals practicing a vegetarian diet has increased over the last decade. Many men and women have converted to a plant-based diet for various reasons whether it was because they felt sympathy for farm animals, they themselves have had a series of health issues that require an immediate intervention, they want to get away from growth hormones and other toxins found in animal products, because they realize the benefits of a plant-based diet in the long run, or in many cases, it is a combination of all of the above. Whatever one's reason for going vegetarian, he/she has chosen a very beneficial path to say the least.

Now that many people have chosen a plant-based diet, the question arises, one that I get from friends, family, and strangers all too often, "Where do I start?" This is a question filled with just as much enthusiasm as there is confusion. Most of us would really like to make that change but we just don't know where to begin. Fortunately, that question alone has been the key motivating factor for this book as I will clearly and concisely expound on the transitioning process to a vegetarian diet for those seeking direction.

*Note: For the sake of clarity and confusion, the focus in this short reading will be for those who are seeking a vegetarian diet as opposed to a vegan diet--I will explain the difference of the two later.

The Link between Red/Processed Meat and Cancer

On Monday, October 26, 2015 The International Agency for Research on Cancer, *IARC* (the cancer agency of the World Health Organization, *WHO*) announced the consumption of red and processed meat causes cancer. "The most influen-tial evidence came from large prospective cohort studies conducted over the past 20 years" the report stated. It has been well-known for decades that processed and red-meat causes cancer, but I guess most people just didn't believe the hype. Within the *wholistic* community, meat that has been processed or meat that contains growth hormones (as most meat produced today does), arsenic, and other dangerous chemicals is one of the leading contributors to cancer.

What exactly is processed meat? The report gives a working definition of just what processed meat is: "meat that has been transformed through salting, curing, fermentation, smoking, or other processes to enhance flavour or improve preservation. Most processed meats contain pork or beef, but processed meats may also contain other red meats, poultry, offal, or meat by-products such as blood." The report goes on to define red-meat as, "all types of mammalian muscle meat, such as beef, veal, pork, lamb, mutton, horse, and goat." The agency even went as far as to give a short list of foods that cause cancer naming such foods as: hot dogs, sausages, ham, corned-beef, and beef jerky.

Upon observing this report, one would assume that because chicken or fish was not mentioned that it may be safe to consume. The problem with this is that unless one is raising his/her own chickens or fish and can supervise what these animals are being fed day-to-day, he/she truly does not know if these animals have been fed any cancer causing substances; so yes, even fish and chicken should be looked at under a microscope for those who once believed that chicken and fish were safe.

Now or Never

With the announcement of the health risks of processed meat and the thousands of new incidences of cancer and other serious health conditions each year, a new approach to how we eat is definitely in order. Now that it has been made official that these meats cause cancer, this is the perfect time to choose an alternative, and that alternative is a plant-based diet. You have made it this far by opening up the front cover and dedicating some time to reading the words that have been written so it is safe to say that if you haven't made up your mind to commit to a vegetarian diet 100% then you are very close! With that being said, allow me to be your guide on this journey to a new, healthier, way of living.

Chapter One

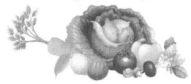

What is a Vegetarian?

"Nothing tastes as good as being healthy feels." – Unknown.

The Merriam-Webster dictionary defines a vegetarian as - "a person who does not eat meat" or "consisting wholly of vegetables, fruits, grains, nuts, and sometimes eggs or dairy products" – I personally prefer the latter over the first definition. This is the technical description of vegetarianism which is widely accepted, however, I want to present my own definition of what a vegetarian is: a vegetarian is someone whose diet consists primarily of fruits, vegetables, nuts/grains, and consumes dairy products infrequently while overall training themselves to become a vegan. Yup, that's right. My definition of a vegetarian is pretty much someone who is in training to become a vegan. Remember all of those reasons I mentioned earlier, as far as why individuals convert to a vegetarian diet? Well, *most* of those actually are not satisfied by a vegetarian diet, but by a vegan diet, however, I realize we have to take it one step at a time just as I did when I finally made the decision.

Vegan vs. Vegetarian

One thing that I often come across is confusion on the differences between a vegetarian and a vegan diet because many believe that both are the same thing. As mentioned earlier, a vegetarian is someone who does not eat meat and primarily has a diet of fruits, veggies, nuts, grains, and dairy products. A vegan on the other hand is an individual who does not *consume* or utilize *anything* that comes from an animal, big difference; vegetarians eat cheese/eggs, drink milk, and may use or wear products made from animals (leather, fur coats, etc.), vegans do not eat eggs/cheese, drink cow's milk, or wear any product that has come from an animal or has been tested on an animal.

Benefits of a Vegetarian Diet

A plant-based diet has many benefits that can include: clearer skin, a slimmer waist and sto-mach, mild to significant weight loss, not to mention the more tolerable aroma after one handles their business in the bathroom amongst many other things. Dr. Michael Klaper's presentation of *Foods That Kill* (available on YouTube) dives deeper into the internal benefits of a plant-based diet. The presentation, just as relevant and beneficial now as it was back in 1993, provides us with Dr. Klaper's first-hand experience with those who have chosen to consume meat as their primary source of nutrition versus vegetables. Check it out.

Many of us today, especially black men and women, suffer from high blood pressure--from aunties, to uncles, to mothers and fathers--we all know someone who suffers from this ailment and is medicated with some form of a drug from their doctor as "treatment." With such a prevalent condition, more times than often stemming from one's diet and constantly being in a stressful environment, it is obvious that what we eat plays a major part being that we consume more processed food and meat than ever before. I mean think about it--some of us have had a less than nutritious diet pretty much our entire lives, some health issues are bound to arise eventually and they typically do in our latter years. As Dr. Klaper mentioned in his findings with those who have adopted a vegetarian diet, they were able to slowly but surely get off of their medication and successfully regulated their blood pressure just by switching their diet.

It's that simple, however, regulating blood pressure is not the only benefit. I have personally experienced individuals tell me that they have lower cholesterol (higher counts of HDL and a lower LDL), twice the amount of energy, they feel less toxic and they overall just feel great. A major observation one may immediately be aware of is that they don't feel drained after eating a meal which is known all too well to meat eaters. After eating a large meal, many get the urge to take a nap, better known as the 'itis'; this happens as a result of the high density meal one has just consumed where the body directs most of its attention (energy) to digestion leaving one feeling lethargic.

How Eating Meat is Affecting You, Spiritually

By now you are aware of some of the physical advantages of going vegetarian, but now I would like to view meat consumption and vegetarianism from a spiritual standpoint. Because of industry farming where large quantities of meat have to be produced at a constant and rapid rate, companies raise animals in a very *congested* and *disturbing* way! Animals are treated with little to *no* remorse for their lives, all in the name of a number two at the local fast food joint or a ten-piece wing ding at the restaurant down the street. Because these animals are raised in such a way, they are constantly filled with pain, anguish, fear, and are extremely stressed amongst other fear based emotions (yes animals have emotions and can be stressed). So, the question is, "How does this affect the person who eats these animals?"

When one eats meat (meat that has been raised on an industrial farm), because of the way in which these animals are killed and slaughtered during the "preparation process", the stress, fear, and every other emotion (emotion, e-motion=energy in motion) that the animal felt at the point of death is transferred during consumption. The same stress and fear that that cow or chicken felt while being butchered is nothing more than energy, and we all know from physics class that energy can never be destroyed only transferred and transformed--so what do you think happens when one eats the flesh of that animal? That energy is transferred and assimilated into their being.

Have you ever been in a room with a friend or someone whose vibe was just off and you noticed it began to rub off on you? Imagine the same thing happening, but from the inside out. Imagine how this is affecting you in the now and in ten to twenty years. Also take into consideration that, unless there is an underlying medical condition, *excessive* weight gain is an indication of high levels of stress within the body. Excessive weight is an aggregation of energy--an energy of stress. I can almost guarantee that individuals who are deemed obese are mentally/emotionally stressed. One must ask his/herself, "Whose stress am I carrying around, my own or that of the dearly departed?" Eating is a form of communication, we must be conscious of what we're telling our body.

The Vegetarian Myth

When we hear of someone who is vegetarian, our minds have been conditioned to instantly assume that that individual "only eats salads." Back when I was vegetarian, this was the most common response I got from friends and strangers, and you will probably experience the same. In the black community, while there are quite a few vegetarians amongst us, they are scattered about. Because of this, when we do come across someone who is vegetarian it's like we just found Big-Foot. We are so intrigued by their choice of diet that we ask them question after question as if they're from another planet.

What we don't realize when it comes to being a vegetarian is that just because one does not eat meat anymore does not automatically make he or she healthy. One can be vegetarian and *still* eat unhealthy every single day; cheese pizza, mozzarella sticks, candy, potato chips, pies, ice-cream, TV-dinners, the list goes on and on. The goal to becoming vegetarian is not simply the avoidance of meat, the goal is to adopt a *plant-based* diet rich in fruit, vegetables, nuts, seeds, and grains. Don't become the vegetarian who actually turns out to be unhealthier than they were when they ate meat.

Chapter Two

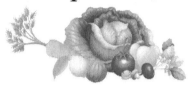

The Elimination Process

~2~

Going from eating meat to becoming a vegetarian has its many paths. Some of us have to take it slow, while others can wake up one day and completely call it quits, never eating a piece of meat ever again. No *one* process is the "right" way to go about transitioning. Find whatever works for you and focus on that. We all have different drives and motivations so don't allow someone else's journey to force you into a process that makes you uncomfortable in yours – to each his or her own.

Transitioning

When it comes to changing something you've done your entire life, it is best to give yourself time to adjust to the new lifestyle. The most common way of going vegetarian is to slowly start eliminating different meats one-by-one unless you're like the minority and can go cold-turkey. Below is an example of how you can go about the elimination process, it can be done weekly or bi-weekly, which ever works best for you. Keep in mind that although each week a different item is eliminated you don't have to eliminate *that specific* item during any given week. You very well may find it more suitable for you to eliminate beef or seafood during week one instead of pork and so on.

- ❖ Stage 1(Week 1) – Eliminate pork – This is the initiation stage. Here you may have doubts that you can do it or you may second guess yourself about becoming a vegetarian but stick with it, this is the second most difficult stage. I say it is the second most difficult stage because usually in the first stage people give up the meat that they like the least however, getting over the mental conditioning of eating meat which may have been present from very early on tends to be the most difficult at the beginning. The last stage typically is the most difficult but certainly *not* impossible. Once you have a solid grip on managing the cravings you may get for pork products, you are now ready to move on to the second stage.

❖ Stage 2(Week 2) – Eliminate beef – In stage two the momentum is shifting and you may be feeling more confident in your transition. As with pork, once you have a solid grip on managing the cravings you may get for beef, you are now ready to move on to the third stage.

❖ Stage 3(Week 3) – Eliminate seafood – By the time you reach the third stage you have built up momentum and you are getting the hang of a life without meat. You have eliminated a few of the foods that you have eaten for quite a long time and fought off the cravings along the way—even if you may have had one or two slip ups but you got back on track, that's cool too, there's absolutely nothing wrong with that. At this point you start to feel confident in your ability and discipline. Once you have mastered this stage you are now ready to move on to the final stage.

❖ Stage 4(Week 4) – Eliminate chicken –In the last stage, transitioning vegetarians usually hold on to the food that they love and are addicted to the most saving it as the last thing that they give up. From experience, typically that food is either chicken or seafood. Here you are right on the cusp of becoming a full blown vegetarian (that's if you only ate pork, beef, seafood, and chicken. If you have a more extensive carnivorous diet, then your process may be a bit longer). Once you have given up chicken or whatever that last piece of meat is for you, you begin to see the light! You've been at it for weeks now and have displayed discipline and commitment to your health. It's not easy giving up something you've done your entire life; be proud of your discipline. After a few weeks, once you have given up that last piece of meat and you have adopted more fruits and vegetables into your diet, you may notice that you don't feel tired after meals and you actually feel lighter in weight and spirit. You are now a vegetarian!

*Note: In the process above, I have broken it down to four stages, however, depending on your eating habits you may have to add or subtract weeks/stages to your process.

Cravings

Cravings come from addictive foods; foods that have been genetically modified and contain chemicals or foods that contain large quantities of sugar. *Real* food does not addict. One cannot be addicted to an apple or lettuce because these foods do not create an energetic deficit within the body. Addiction and cravings come in when what one eats has taxed the body of vital energy and instead of providing the body with nutrients; it requires more energy from the body to be digested which creates an imbalance. Eating is a give and take formula. The object of eating is to put back what has been lost. When one consumes dead, putre-fied, and overcooked meat, that meat has been devitalized almost entirely so it cannot give the body what it needs upon consumption, therefore it taxes the body and gives little in return. Digestion uses a lot of energy which is why when we eat heavy meals we get sleepy. The body is diverting its attention (energy) to the process of digestion which causes other bodily functions to seemingly "shut down".

When it comes to dealing with cravings one way to curve them is to eat something healthy (trail mix, fruit, a salad, etc.) until the sensation has diminished. Cravings can drive us crazy but the good thing is that they don't last forever. The longer we refrain from eating that bacon, seafood, or chicken we're craving, the less sever the cravings become until they completely disappear. Some cravings may take longer than others to go away, but they will go away.

Chapter Three

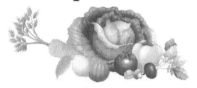

Becoming a Complete Vegetarian

~3~

"A healthy body is the only vehicle that will make us realize our Godliness." – Llaila O. Afrika

We all have our own path to a healthy lifestyle but along the way there can be certain factors or pieces of information that act as a catalyst. Witnessing a family member struggle with their health and go through a near-death experience can definitely catapult us to leave certain foods or lifestyles alone. This is exactly what sparked my curiosity in vegetarianism. Years ago when I was an undergrad in college in Nashville, TN, I received a call from my sister who told me what had happened back home. It turned out that my father underwent mitral valve repair where heart surgeons went in and repaired a leaking heart valve; basically, open-heart surgery. It was a tough time to say the least. Anyone in their right mind who goes through a situation like that will begin to do some introspection of their own and begin to eliminate the things in their life (negative thoughts/emotions, unhealthy foods, stressful relationships, etc.) that are unhealthy out of fear of something similar happening to them.

As if this wasn't enough, *shortly* after my father's operation, my mother fell sick in which she had to undergo surgery where doctors removed a tumor from her brain. Scary right? This added insult to injury because prior to this operation, my mother was diagnosed with thyroid cancer where she had to have her thyroid gland completely removed. I'm glad to say she is a survivor of both operations today and both of my parents are doing better.

This is just an example of how certain life situations can lead to drastic lifestyle changes. When a family member has a serious health crisis, always look at the underlying issue because a good percentage of the time it is due to spiritual/emotional/nutritional related imbalances.

Modern medicine may have us believe certain diseases "run in a family" (ex. diabetes and obesity), but this is false. Obesity and diabetes do not run in a family, but the eating habits that cause obesity and diabetes do. An entire family may be overweight because they all eat the same, not because of genetics. Anyone in opposition to this fact should study the science of *Epigenetics*.

There Isa good-deal of documentaries that also act as catalysts in helping one convert to a plant-based diet. They give the raw uncut truth on industry farming and how "farm" animals are raised and butchered for profit. A few of these titles include: *Lucent, Cowspiracy*, and *Food, Inc.* There are other titles that look to simply educate individuals on the benefits of a vegetarian diet and the deleterious effects of a diet predominately centered on animal flesh. These titles include: *Soul Food Junkies, Forks Over Knives, Vegucated, Hungry for Change, Fat, Sick, & Nearly Dead, Food Matters*, and *GMO OMG*. I recommend checking these titles out as they will give you great knowledge on the subject. Most, if not all of these titles are available on Netflix or YouTube.

<u>Critics</u>

As with anything that is an anomaly or different from the "normal" flow of things in the public eye, you will experience critics. The stricter the diet and the more things you begin to eliminate, the more criticism you will come across. Most criticism will come from family members with friends coming in a close second. Food is seemingly held to the same standard as religion. One grows up eating a certain way and as he/she gets older this pattern is continued unquestioned. When one breaks away from the way his/her family does things and it gets to the point where family members can see a change in eating habits, the questions and slick comments start. Imagine someone who grew up Christian and at the age of nineteen they decide to learn about other religions that satisfied their needs better, their family may begin to feel a certain type of way. Some members of the family might even start to feel as if he/she thinks they are "better" than them; which is not the case at all, it's just that they have begun to question the status quo instead of simply going along with it. There's absolutely nothing wrong with seeking a lifestyle that best fits you.

Stick with It

A great way to maintain a certain way of eating is to surround yourself with friends and family members who eat the same way as you do, if at all possible. The habits of others can rub off on us if we're not careful or disciplined enough in our practice. Surround yourself with friends who are either already vegetarian/vegan or who are also making the transition – trust me, it makes life much easier. You both can trade new information that you've found, recipes, or stories about how you stopped eating certain types of meat and other unhealthy foods. It's just like if you were looking to become an artist; you would surround yourself with other likeminded artists that will inspire, motivate, and guide you. If you don't have any friends or family members that live a plant-based lifestyle or are at least in the process of doing so, create one (haha). Ask your mother, or father, or best friend if he/she has ever thought about living out a healthier life. Explain the benefits to them, show them one of the documentaries mentioned earlier, give them an incentive to want to at least try it out, you never know, you may change someone's life.

Health Benefits

The benefits of a plant-based diet touch every aspect of our health. This is especially apparent in the realm of chronic ailments. Chronic illnesses are illnesses that are long term: arthritis, congestive heart failure, hypothyroidism, hyperthyroidism, etc. A plant-based diet is well known for its ability to reverse chronic illnesses. There are many cases of individuals who converted to a plant-based diet, consuming more fruits and vegetables, and they were able to cut-back on their medication and quite often they were able to completely get off of it! There are copious stories of individuals who had high blood pressure or high cholesterol and after going vegetarian they were able to get their readings back within range. These individuals supplemented those synthetic, overly expensive, highly toxic pharmaceutical drugs for fruit and veggies. That sounds like a fair trade to me.

Chapter Four

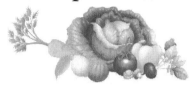

Shopping for Fruits and Veggies

~4~

"People eat meat thinking they will become as strong as an ox, forgetting that the ox eats grass."

– Pino Caruso

When shopping for fruits and vegetables it is better to purchase from a local farmer's market in your area, but if this is not possible, go with the next best selection available (ex. a grocery store). When purchasing fruit and vegetables from a grocery store, check the package or label for the location of where the produce was grown. Packages are usually labeled with the state in which the fruit came from – look for produce grown in your state *if possible* and *when applicable* (keeping in mind that certain fruits are grown in certain climates and locations) and always go organic whenever possible.

Eating at Restaurants

A common question that I get is "What do you eat when you go to restaurants?" whenever I find myself at a restaurant and the menu isn't vegetarian friendly, I improvise. For example, I may order a chicken salad and tell the waitress to hold off on the chicken and add more veggies or I may order certain pastas without meat and add mushrooms and onions. It's fairly easy to work around eating meat at restaurants, you just have to do a little adding or subtracting. I find that at the very least, restaurants have veggie burger substitutes for most of the burgers they offer on their menu. The types of patties that are offered as substitutes are sometimes located in small print near the bottom of the column of burgers to choose from. The most common are black bean or quinoa burgers.

Meal Creativity

Be creative with your meals. There are endless possibilities and variations of vegetarian meals to choose from. One good way to get going and develop your arsenal of vegetarian recipes is to purchase a vegetarian cookbook. My favorite book to choose recipes from is, "A Taste of Life: 1,000 Vegetarian Recipes from Around the World" by Dr. Supreme Understanding. There are many fulfilling meals to choose from as a vegetarian, the object is to familiarize yourself with what's out there. I've used google on several occasions to explore the different possibilities; the information is out there you just have to do a little research.

Juicing/Smoothies

Juicing has become increasingly popular as more individuals incorporate more fruits and vegetables into their diet. Juicing has its benefits. The digestion process converts whatever we eat into a liquid and it is then absorbed through the intestinal wall. When we juice however, this process is cut in half because we've already converted our food into liquid form. The fruit or veggie juice/smoothieis digested and easily moves through our system with less energy being expended giving our bodies what it needs much faster. It is digested much quicker than if we were to eat a solid meal.

This dynamic partly explains why when we eat heavy meals we get the *itis*. When we eat a heavy meal and we get sleepy afterwards, what is happening is our body has converged a large amount of energy to the digestion process so that it can breakdown everything that was just eaten as mentioned earlier in the book. As a result of energy being redirected, our bodies seemingly shut-down and we immediately get tired or sleepy. It makes sense when one thinks about it; to get an idea of how hard the body has to work, just imagine the effort involved in turning a solid steak into a liquid. A list of smoothie recipes can be found in Appendix II.

Chapter Five

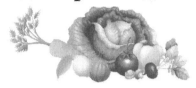

The Final Steps

~5~

"When the ears of the student are ready to hear, then come the lips to fill them with wisdom."
- The Kybalion

As you begin to grow and explore new healthy recipes or bear witness to the health advantages that are associated with a plant-based diet, it is likely that your initial reaction will be to share your experience with friends and family, and you should! As you become more knowledgeable about the vegetarian lifestyle, reach out and help those who are seeking the path themselves. Share recipes with them, tell them about your personal experiences as you transitioned from eating meat; share this book with them - anything to aide in their process. It is much easier to break a habit or transition to a new lifestyle when we have other people in our lives that can give us advice, motivate us, or tell us stories of their experiences. Each one, teach one.

Exercising to Increase Benefits

We all know the benefits of exercise, but when exercise is combined with a plant-based diet, rather vegan or vegetarian, the benefits are multiplied. Your body looks more toned, you feel lighter, and overall you have more energy. Many of us believe that without eating animal flesh we won't have enough energy, or that we won't get the proper amount of protein needed to re-build muscles. Nothing could be further from the truth! There are plenty of vegetables with high concentrations of protein such as:

- Broccoli
- Peas
- Lentils
- Asparagus
- Spinach
- Kale
- Brussels Sprouts
- Artichokes

Don't believe the hype when it comes to the myth that you absolutely need to consume meat to build muscle and get stronger. There are plenty of professional athletes who are either vegan or vegetarian. One example we can look at to combat this myth is Chicago Bears' defensive tackle David Carter who is a vegan. Here we have a professional NFL player weighing 300lbs and can perform at a high level. There are many other athletes doing the same; from body-builders, to tennis and baseball players. Every time a professional athlete who eats a plant-based diet performs, the lack of protein myth gets buried deeper and deeper.

Becoming a Vegan

As mentioned earlier, a vegan and vegetarian diet are two completely different things. When it comes to pursuing a vegan diet, the commonly traveled path is to go vegetarian initially, then convert over to veganism. There are individuals who can make the transition from eating meat and dairy to becoming a full blown vegan; it's a rare occurrence but it does happen. This type of transition takes a tremendous amount of discipline. You will probably hear many people make the claim that they've up and gone vegan throughout your journey, only to hear later on down the line how they just finished eating a steak, I've heard it plenty of times. Many people try to sprint before they even crawl.

Once you feel that you have mastered the art of being a vegetarian, you are now ready to make the second transition to veganism if you choose to do so. Because you traveled the road of vegetarianism first, the transition won't be as harsh had you just up and made the transition directly from eating meat. Just like with a vegetarian diet, there are benefits. There is no time limit to making the transition; some of us can do it in six months, others, six years. It is solely based on how you feel. It took me about two years of being a vegetarian to make the transition to veganism. Everyone has their own path, none greater than the other. In part two of this book, I will assist individuals who are looking to make this transition.

Vitamins and Supplements

One of the main focuses while practicing a plant-based diet, whether *pescatarian* or an *lacto-ovo vegetarian*, is vitamin deficiency. Individuals following a plant-based diet typically have a vitamin B12 deficiency as this vitamin is not found in many fruit and vegetables. Vitamin B12 is well known for helping the body convert the food one has consumed into energy, therefore, after transitioning to a vegetarian diet if you experience a lack of energy, lethargy, weakness, or if you find it more difficult to recall information, more than likely you have a B12 deficiency. This is typically taken care of by incorporating vitamins of the B-complex into your daily diet. Zinc, Iron, and EFAs (essential fatty acids) are on the list of vitamin deficiencies for those who are on a plant-based diet as well. Just as with B12, these vitamins can be supplemented.

*Getting blood work done is a definitive answer for vitamin deficiency. Consult with your physician before taking any vitamin supplements. The information presented above is to be used as a recommendation and not as a substitute for a doctor's advice.

You've Made a Big Step

Deciding to adopt a plant-based diet is no small task. It takes discipline, tenacity, and confidence. You have made the conscious effort to incorporate a better diet into your life and as a result, an increase in your quality of living. Be proud of your accomplishment. Your body will thank you in so many ways and the long-lasting effects of a vege-tarian diet are worth the hard work you've put in. Now your obligation is to share your experience with others who may seek your advice. Once others see how great you look and your posts on social media about your achievements, *many* people will seek your consultation and want to know exactly what you did. Share your experience with friends/family. Your dedication to a better lifestyle will inspire others to do the same. You will be an example of what others can do with hard work and dedication! You've made a big step.

5-Day Meal Plan

A big problem with individuals who are considering a plant-based diet is they simply don't know what to eat – in understanding that, I have incorporated a sample five-day meal plan to give an idea of different meals one can eat. The recipes for the meal plan can be found in Appendix I. Appendix II contains six smoothie recipes, a list of cookbooks, and additional vegetarian recipes.

*****

Day 1

Breakfast: Fruit - kiwi, pineapple, and strawberries
Lunch: Baked sweet potato and salad
Dinner: Black Bean/Butternut Squash Chili *recipe in Appendix I*

Day 2

Breakfast: Whole grain oats with fruit
Lunch: Vegetable wrap
Dinner: Pasta w/Fresh Tomatoes & Basil *recipe in Appendix I*

Day 3

Breakfast: Fruit - (can be eaten whole or turned into a smoothie) strawberry, blueberry, blackberry, and a banana

Lunch: Strawberry and Avocado Spinach Salad with Candid Pecans *recipe in Appendix I*
Dinner: Stuffed Mushrooms *recipe in Appendix I*

Day 4

Breakfast: Fruit - honeydew, watermelon, and cantaloupe
Lunch: Spinach and Mushroom Soup *recipe in Appendix I*
Dinner: Pasta Primavera *recipe in Appendix I*

Day 5

Breakfast: Mixed berry smoothie
Lunch: Spinach salad
Dinner: Vegetable stir fry

Here are some snacks that can be eaten in between meals or in replace of whole meals.

Snacks: raw cashews, guacamole w/ tortilla chips, raw almonds, trail mix, hummus with crackers, fruit, granola bar, crackers with almond butter, cucumbers or celery with dressing, bagel, a muffin, steamed artichoke

Appendix I

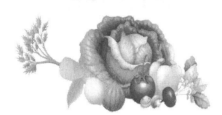

Black Bean/Butternut Squash Chili

-Ingredients-

1 small butternut squash, peeled and cubed

2-3 cups black beans (cooked or canned)

1 onion

Chopped spices – garlic, chili powder, cilantro, cumin, etc.

tomatoes

1 lime, zest and juice

Chipotle peppers (canned, with adobo sauce)

-Cooking Instructions-

1. Sautee onion in small amount of oil until limp.
2. Add chopped garlic and spices and let cook for a few minutes.
3. Add grated zest of lime and squash cubes, cook for about 10 minutes.
4. Add beans, tomatoes, water (if needed), and as many chipotle peppers (they're hot!!).
5. Cook until the squash is tender, at least a half hour.
6. Serve with cilantro and lime juice.

Spinach and Mushroom Soup

-Ingredients-

1 quart vegetable broth

1 cup whole-wheat pasta - Rotelle or other small shaped pasta

1 cup frozen green peas

2 cups baby spinach

3/4 cup mushrooms, quartered

1/2 teaspoon kosher salt

ground black pepper

4 tablespoons shredded parmesan cheese

-Cooking Instructions-

1.   Bring vegetable broth to a boil in a medium saucepan.

2.   Once boiling, add pasta and cook for 5 to 6 minutes

3.   Add peas, spinach and mushrooms, season with salt and pepper and continue to cook for an additional 2 to 3 minutes.

4.   Serve topped with Parmesan cheese.

Pasta w/Fresh Tomatoes & Basil

-Ingredients-

3 tomatoes, seeded and chopped

2 cloves garlic, minced

2 tablespoons chopped fresh parsley

2 tablespoons chopped fresh basil

2 tablespoons lemon juice

½ teaspoon sugar

½ teaspoon salt

¼ teaspoon pepper

¼ olive oil

8 ounces fettuccine pasta, cooked

-Cooking Instructions-

1.   Sautee first 8 ingredients in hot oil in a large skillet over low heat, stirring constantly, 1 minute or until thoroughly heated.

2.   Spoon over hot cooked pasta.

Pasta Primavera

-Ingredients-

3 carrots, peeled and cut into thin strips

2 medium zucchini or 1 large zucchini, cut into thin strips

2 yellow squash, cut into thin strips

1 onion, thinly sliced

1 yellow bell pepper, cut into thin strips

1 red bell pepper, cut into thin strips

1/4 cup olive oil

kosher salt and ground black pepper

1 tablespoon dried Italian herbs

1lb farfalle (bowtie pasta)

15 cherry tomatoes, halved

1/2 cup grated parmesan

-Cooking Instructions-

1. Preheat the oven to 450 degrees F.

2. On a large heavy baking sheet, toss all of the vegetables with the oil, salt, pepper, and dried herbs to coat. Transfer half of the vegetable mixture to another heavy large baking sheet and arrange evenly over the baking sheets. Bake until the carrots are

tender and the vegetables begin to brown, stirring after the first 10 minutes, about 20 minutes total.

3. Meanwhile, cook the pasta in a large pot of boiling salted water until al dente, tender but still firm to the bite, about 8 minutes. Drain but reserve 1 cup of the cooking liquid.

4. Toss the pasta with the vegetable mixtures in a large bowl to combine. Toss with the cherry tomatoes and enough reserved cooking liquid to moisten.

Season the pasta with salt and pepper, to taste. Sprinkle with the Parmesan and serve immediately.

Stuffed Mushrooms

-Ingredients-
12 whole fresh mushrooms
1 tablespoon extra-virgin olive oil
1 tablespoon minced garlic
1 (8 ounce) package cream cheese, softened
$\frac{1}{4}$ cup grated parmesan cheese
$\frac{1}{4}$ teaspoon ground black pepper
$\frac{1}{4}$ teaspoon onion powder
$\frac{1}{4}$ teaspoon ground cayenne pepper

-Cooking Instructions-

1.   Preheat oven to 350 degrees F. Spray baking sheet with cooking spray. Clean mushrooms with a damp paper towel. Carefully break off stems. Chop stems extremely fine, discarding tough end of stems.

2.   Heat oil in a large skillet over medium heat. Add garlic and chopped mushroom stems to the skillet. Fry until any moisture has disappeared, making sure not to burn garlic. Set aside to cool.

3.   When garlic and mushroom mixture is no longer hot, stir in cream cheese, Parmesan cheese, black pepper, onion powder and cayenne pepper. Mixture should be very thick. Using a little spoon,

fill each mushroom cap with a generous amount of stuffing. Arrange the mushroom caps on prepared cookie sheet.

4.   Bake for 20 minutes or until the mushrooms are piping hot and liquid starts to form under caps.

Strawberry and Avocado Spinach Salad with Candied Pecans

-Ingredients-
6 cups baby spinach
2 cups strawberries, stems removed and sliced
1 ripe large avocado, diced
1 teaspoon lemon juice
1/4 cup crumbled feta cheese
2 tablespoons butter
1 cup pecan halves
2 tablespoons brown sugar

-Cooking Instructions-
1.   On the stovetop over medium heat, melt the butter. Stir in the pecan halves until completely incorporated. Stir in the brown sugar and continue to stir until the nuts are fragrant and the sugar is sticking.
2.   Remove from the stovetop and spread evenly on a wax paper-lined baking sheet to dry.
3.   Remove the stems of the strawberries and slice. Remove the peel and pit of the avocado. Chop the avocado and then mix with the lemon juice to avoid browning.
4.   Toss the strawberries and avocado with the spinach.
5.   Stir in the feta cheese and dried candied pecans.
6.   Enjoy.

Appendix II

(More Vegetarian and Smoothie Recipes)

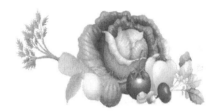

Philly Cheese "Steak"

-Ingredients-
1 tablespoon olive oil
1 medium red onion (sliced thinly)
1 green bell pepper (sliced thinly)
20 ounces of baby Bella mushrooms (sliced)
¼ black pepper
¼ steak season
¼ nature season
¼ dale season
Swiss-cheese
Submarine bread

-Cooking Instructions-
1. Preheat oven to 350 degrees.
2. Add olive oil to medium-heat skillet.
3. Add onion, bell pepper, and mushrooms.
4. Add black pepper, steak season, nature season, and dale season.
5. Let cook for about 15-20 minutes.
6. Place sub bread on cookie sheet, add onion, bell pepper, mushrooms, and cheese to sub.

7. Place in oven until cheese has melted.

8. Add any condiments that you like ex. banana peppers, jalapeno peppers, mayo, mustard, etc.

Veggie Quesadilla

-Ingredients-

1 tablespoon olive oil

½ red onion

½ yellow, red, orange bell pepper

10 ounces Baby bella mushrooms

¼ black pepper

¼ red pepper

¼ nature season

¼ basil

1 cup Mexican blend shredded cheese

2 wheat tortilla

-Cooking Instructions-

1. Place olive oil in medium-heat skillet. *If you do not have a quesadilla-maker, using a round skillet will work just fine.

2. Lightly steam or sauté onion, peppers, mushrooms, black pepper, red pepper, nature seasoning, and basil in skillet.

3. In a separate skillet over medium-heat, pour in a spoon-full of olive oil and place one tortilla on skillet.

4. Add steamed or sautéed veggies and cheese then place other tortilla on top.

5. Use a spatula to flip (cook on each side about 5 minutes).

6. Serve with sour cream, salsa, and lettuce.

Lasagna Rolls

-Ingredients-
3 tsp Basil (dried)
3 Garlic cloves
1 medium Onion
2 tsp Oregano (dried)
2 tsp Parsley (dried)
1 pack Spinach (fresh)
1 can of tomato sauce
salt and pepper
1 tbsp. Olive oil
½ cup Mozzarella cheese
2/3 cup Parmesan cheese
5 oz. Ricotta cheese
12 Wheat lasagna noodles

-Cooking Instructions-
1. Boil lasagna noodles.
2. Mix spinach, mozzarella, parmesan, and ricotta
cheese together in a bowl.
3. Heat sauce pan to low-medium, then sauté
onions with garlic cloves until onions are light

brown then add tomato sauce, oregano, parsley,
and basil then simmer for 20 minutes.

4. Once noodles are tender lay them on wax paper
or a flat surface, then take the spinach and cheeses
and spread across noodles, then roll noodle until
spinach and cheese is in the center of the noodle.

5. Take a baking dish and pour half of the tomato
sauce on the bottom of the dish, then take each
rolled noodle and place them on top of tomato
sauce, finally, take the other half of tomato sauce
and cover the top half of the noodles and top with
mozzarella cheese.

6. Bake in oven for 25 minutes.

7. Enjoy.

Mushroom Pasta

-Ingredients-

16 ounces fresh mushroom, halved

3 cloves garlic, minced

3 tablespoons olive oil

2/3 cups dry white wine

4 to 5 plum tomatoes, cut into chunks

½ cups green onions, sliced

½ cups firmly packed fresh basil leaves

½ teaspoon salt or to taste

¾ teaspoon freshly ground pepper

8 ounces spaghetti, cooked

-Cooking instructions-

1. Sauté mushrooms and garlic in hot oil in a large skillet for 4 minutes or until tender.

2. Add wine and bring to boil.

3. Boil, stirring occasionally, 6 minutes or until mixture is reduced by half.

4. Stir in tomato, green onions, and next 3 ingredients.

5. Cook, stirring occasionally, until thoroughly heated.

6. Spoon over hot cooked pasta.

<u>Roasted Vegetable Sandwich</u>

-Ingredients-

2 med eggplant

1 zucchini

1 red bell pepper

1 yellow bell pepper

1 yellow onion

1 red onion

1 tablespoon olive oil

3 cloves garlic (change to taste)

fresh basil

-Cooking Instructions-

1. Slice vegetables/finely chop garlic and put into 9x13 pan.

2. Drizzle with olive oil.

3. Place in preheated oven (350-375) and roast for about an hour, turning contents every 15 minutes.

4. Serve on bread with fresh basil *Toast bread for optimal taste.

5. Feel free to add cheese.

Smoothies

Smoothies are great in the morning because they are made within 5-10 minutes and give the body a boost of energy to begin the day. They do not require as much energy to digest like a solid breakfast would (ex. eggs, toast, sausage, etc.) because of their liquid form – leaving you feeling vitalized and ready to start your day. I recommend limiting the use of ice as ice shocks the body's digestive system due to its cold temperature throwing off the digestive process. Use ice only when absolutely necessary or in small amounts.

Blueberry Green Smoothie

-Ingredients-

2 cups water

1 cup spinach

1 ½ cups fresh blueberries

1 banana

1 tablespoon EFA oil

2 tablespoons agave nectar

-Instructions-

1. Place ingredients into blender.

2. Blend it for about 1 minute or until spinach is completed mixed.

<u>Very Berry</u>

-Ingredients-

½ cup blueberries

½ cup blackberries

½ cup strawberries

1 banana

½ cup almond milk

-Instructions-

1. Add blueberries and blackberries.

2. Cut up strawberries and banana and add to mix.

3. Pour in almond milk and blend.

Granola – Almond Butter Crunch

-Ingredients-

1 cup of granola

1 banana

½ cup of Almond Butter (a peanut butter substitute)

½ blueberries

1 cup of almond milk (or until desired thickness is
reached)

2-3 cubes of ice

-Instructions-

1. Chop up banana and add it to mixing cup along
with almond butter and blueberries.

2. Pour in granola then add almond milk and ice.

3. Mix for 1 minute then check mix for thickness –
add more almond milk as needed.

4. Mix again for 1 minute.

<u>Citrus Blast</u>

-Ingredients-

2 kiwis

1 cup of pineapple

1 orange

½ cup of water

-Instructions-

1. Mix all of the ingredients for about 1 minute.

Pina Colada

-Ingredients-
1 cup coconut milk
½ frozen banana
1 cup fresh pineapple
1 tablespoon honey

-Instructions-
1. Freeze banana and pineapple overnight in a freezer bag.
2. Put all ingredients in blender together.
3. Blend until smooth.
4. Pour into tall glass and top with whip cream and cherry.

Spinach Smoothie

-Ingredients-

2 cups of spinach

½ banana

½ to ¾ cups of frozen pineapple

¼ to ½ cup water (depending on desired thickness)

-Instructions-

1. Throw everything in a blender and blend for about a minute.

2. If using frozen pineapple, you should make sure that this is closest to the blade so that it blends well.

3. After a while, you'll probably wean yourself off of needing the pineapple. But if you do, you may want to start freezing bananas to get that consistency the frozen fruit adds.

Vegetarian Cookbooks

*Some vegan cookbooks may be used to make vegetarian
meals also*

- A Taste of life: 1,000 Vegetarian Recipes from Around the World
- Vegan Soul Kitchen: Fresh, Healthy, and Creative African-American Cuisine
- Forks Over Knives The Cookbook: Over 300 Recipes for Plant-Based Eating All Through the Year
- Afro-Vegan: Farm-Fresh African, Caribbean, and Southern Flavors Remixed
- The Oh She Glows Cookbook: Over 100 Vegan Recipes to Glow from the Inside Out
- But I Could Never Go Vegan!: 125 Recipes That Prove You Can Live Without Cheese, It's Not All Rabbit Food, and Your Friends Will Still Come Over For Dinner
- The Complete Vegetarian Cookbook
- Meatless: More Than 200 of the Very Best Vegetarian Recipes
- Veganomicon: The Ultimate Vegan Cookbook
- Vegan Cookbook for Beginners: The Essential Vegan Cookbook to Get Started

~Notes~

*Use this section to make notes, or document your own
journey to becoming a vegetarian.*